Herbal Remedies & Natural Healing From Your Garden

A Practical Guide to Harness the Power of Plants for Health and Wellness

Olivia Phillips

Contents

Part Four
Building Your Home Apothecary

Introduction

Herbalism is the oldest of medicinal practices. It's the use of plants and plant extracts to treat various ailments and used to be limited to traditional medicines such as traditional Chinese medicine and Ayurvedic. Even in the West, the knowledge of medicinal plants was accumulated by the ancient Greeks and Romans.

Many medicines that are used today stem from natural sources. Aspirin came from willow bark, digitalis from foxglove, opium from poppies, and quinine from the Andean fever tree. The chemical compounds found in plants are generally primary and secondary metabolites. While the primary metabolites are used to keep the plant functioning, the secondary metabolites protect the plant from attack or attract the necessary pollinators. It's the secondary metabolites that are used in alternative medicines in people.

While people in developed countries have access to a range of pharmaceutical drugs, some are returning to the use of herbal remedies due to the side effects often associated with pharmaceutical drugs. However, it's important to remember that the use of herbal remedies is the same as that of other supplements, meaning that they aren't regulated by the Food and Drug Administration (FDA). Because of this, there are less stringent tests done as herbal remedies aren't considered drugs. This can lead to people using herbal remedies unsafely, as they don't know about the possible interactions that can occur when taking herbal supplements with pharmaceutical drugs or other herbal supplements.

While many will say there isn't evidence that herbal remedies are better than pharmaceutical drugs, there is so much anecdotal evidence that tests are being run on many old herbal remedies that are still used today.

History of Herbalism

The exact time when herbalism started is unknown, but it's believed that it started when ancient humans started observing what animals ate and then using trial and error to determine what was good to use for what ailments.

The earliest documentation of ancient humans coming into contact with and using plants is probably between 25000 and 13000 B.C.E. It is unknown if this was a way to document what was edible or what had a medicinal value.

Remnants of yarrow and marshmallow root have been discovered in Stone Age burials in Iraq, showing that ancient humans had placed some form of value on these herbs. There are even ancient texts from ancient Mesopotamia and Egypt that show that various plants were being used to treat an array of ailments. Some hieroglyphs depict the use of senna pods to treat constipation, while caraway and peppermint were used for other digestive issues.

Introduction

It's believed that the knowledge of plant-based remedies was verbally handed down through the ages before they were added to various books. The collection of herbal information was often gathered in what was known as herbal pharmacopoeia. The oldest of these was *Pen Ts'ao* by Shen Nung in roughly 2800 B.C.E. The next oldest was from records obtained by King Hammurabi of Babylon in 1800 B.C.E. and came with an array of instructions to use many medicinal plants.

During the Middle Ages, it was commonplace for families to have a small part of the garden dedicated to the growth of herbs to help with common ailments. Villages and towns would also have an herbalist who trained an apprentice. However, this was a dangerous practice during this time, as the act of herbalism was seen as witchcraft and carried the penalty of death.

Thankfully, during the 1500s, King Henry VIII saw the value in herbal medicine, as he created the Charter of King Henry VIII to help the poor get the necessary treatments when they were ill. This charter also protected the herbalists from prosecution.

During the 17th century, the knowledge of herbal remedies became more widespread, and by 1649, a layman-aimed pharmacopoeia, *The English Physician*, was published by Nicholas Culpeper. Despite this, correctly identifying the medicinal plants was difficult, and it wasn't until the 18th century that Carl von Linné developed his classification system to assist with the identification and naming of organisms. Armed with the correct Latin names, and not just common names, it became easier to identify the correct species of plants required.

Introduction

During the 19th century, it became possible to identify, isolate, extract, and then synthesize the compounds from plants that had been used to treat ailments. In the modern age, people are turning back to herbalism to help them with issues they're having, as they're concerned over side effects that some drugs have.

Health Benefits of Cultivating and Using Herbs

Growing medicinal herbs comes with many benefits—especially if you know which plants can treat different ailments. Depending on which herbs you're growing, you can:

- treat headaches and migraines
- treat stomach and digestive ailments
- boost immunity
- lower stress
- soothe pain
- ease muscle pain
- strengthen respiratory system

Herbs are also full of vital vitamins and minerals while also being high in antioxidants and have antiviral, antibacterial, and antifungal properties. Gardening also comes with an array of benefits from exercise, getting fresh air, and vitamin D. The blossoms from herbs will attract beneficial insects to your garden, which is good news if you have vegetables and fruits growing close by.

How to Use This Guide

Starting a medicinal garden to grow your own herbal remedies isn't only easy but also fun. This book aims to teach you how to:

- create an indoor or outdoor garden
- choose the best herbs for common ailments
- harvest and prepare herbs for later use
- create herbal remedies for common ailments
- slowly build an apothecary over time
- personalize herbal remedies for specific conditions
- so much more

Too many people are rushing to emergency rooms for ailments that can be treated early at home with an array of herbal remedies. As long as the plant used is done so correctly and has no interactions with other plants or medications, making herbal remedies is easy and safe to do. Dive into the wonderful world of herbalism and plant remedies!

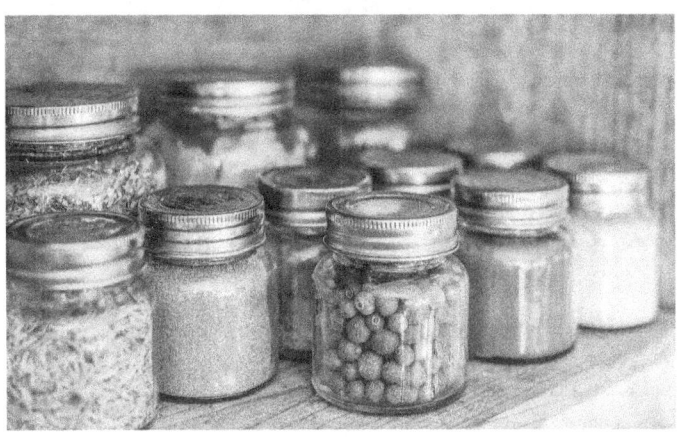

Part One

Fundamentals of Herbal Gardening

In this section, we'll discuss what's needed to have the perfect garden and choose some of the best herbs to grow in your medicinal garden.

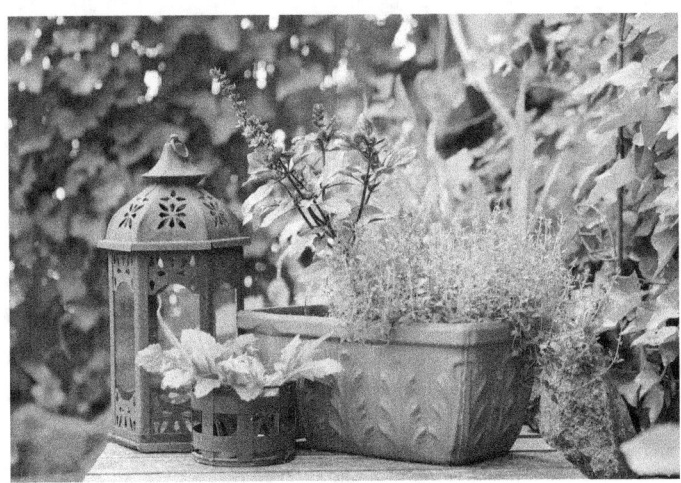

Chapter 1
Fundamentals of Herbal Gardening

The success of your herbal garden depends on you meeting the needs of the plants that are to grow in it and finding the best possible location for them to grow in. Before you can consider planting anything, you need to have the correct area for your plants. When choosing a location, you have to consider the general needs of all plants: water, sunlight, and fertile soil.

A garden and plant layout is dependent on the hemisphere. A garden in the northern hemisphere should run from south to north, with the taller plants planted to the northern side and shorter plants more toward the south. This is the opposite in the southern hemisphere. Growing any garden this way will ensure that all plants get equal sunlight, no matter what time of the day.

Unlike fruiting vegetables and fruits, herbs only require about six hours of sunlight. However, when grown indoors, they require more light with artificial growing lights to get the same duration and strength of light that outdoor plants would get with sunlight.

To determine the best location for maximum sun absorption, spend some time looking at how the sun moves over your property. It's important to note how the shadows move, as not all herbs are tolerant of growing in partial sunlight. Once you have located the perfect area(s) for your herbal garden, note how close it is to a water source. While it's possible to carry water back and forth, it is backbreaking work and shouldn't have to be necessary when a garden is well-planned. It's also important that the location you choose is in a place you can monitor easily. Crops can be quickly destroyed by pests and diseases when not correctly monitored.

The next thing that needs to be looked at is the quality of the soil. Most backyard soils are old and have had most nutrients used up. Low-fertile soils won't produce well. While the soil can be enriched with organic matter and fertilizer, this can take time. The easiest technique to use to avoid extra work is to use a raised garden bed, containers, or permaculture, where fertile soil and organic matter are added to the top of the existing soil, creating a fertile barrier between the plants and the native soil.

Herbal gardens may not be as appealing to pest species as vegetable gardens, but there is a chance that you may have visitors now and again. To avoid this, you can install a fence around the garden to keep out larger herbivores. You can also lay down some landscaping fabric before building your garden to prevent ground-based pests from getting to your crops.

Lastly, you will have to consider the hardiness zone you're in. The hardiness zone will impact when you can grow what is outside, as the first and last frost dates will affect your plants.

Once you have a location in mind, ensure that it isn't in a low-lying area, as this is where water will gather and negatively affect your plants. You will also need to note how wind moves through the area, as you may have to protect your taller plants.

Plant Requirements

Once the location is perfect, you will need to look at the plant's requirements. Different types of plants have different requirements to thrive. Plants have three types of lifecycles. The annuals are plants that complete their entire lifecycle within a year. Biennials generally only develop leaves within the first year of life, while the second is dedicated to creating seeds. Perennials are plants that last several years, producing seeds yearly, but tend to die back or have slowed growth during the colder months. In the lower hardiness zones or where hard frost is an issue, perennials are grown as annuals as the cold kills them.

Herbs require a minimum of six hours of sunlight, but each type may prefer direct sunlight, while others are more comfortable with partial sunlight. When purchasing seeds or seedlings, check the requirements before planting so they are placed in the correct location in your garden.

When it comes to soil, most plants grow at their best in fertile, well-draining, loamy soil, as it's capable of retaining water and nutrients better than other soil types. Poor soils can be amended by working organic matter and fertilizer into it.

It isn't just the type of soil that's important. The pH will affect plants' ability to absorb certain nutrients when not in the correct range. Most plants enjoy a pH range of 6.5–7.5. The pH and fertility of the soil can be tested, though this service can be pricy.

Plants also have space requirements, as seen on seed packets. When placed too close to other plants, there is an excess of competition, causing a failure to thrive. Careful consideration needs to be taken when planting seeds or seedlings, as the full size of the plant may be more than anticipated. Some plants are also aggressive growers and should be contained and not allowed to grow freely.

Lastly, the water needs of plants are not all the same. It may be a good idea to keep water-hungry plants away from those that are more drought-tolerant and don't need as much water. Parsley and basil enjoy moist soil, while thyme and rosemary don't. If the plant's requirements aren't met, it will fail to thrive.

Growing Indoors or Outdoors

Whether growing indoors or outdoors, plants will need extra care. Each has pros and cons, and which you decide to do will depend on the space you have and how much time and money you're willing to invest.

Growing indoors	Growing outdoors
• not affected by hardiness zones	• affected by hardiness zones
• limited space and requires containers	• not as limited by space
• may require artificial lights, especially during the colder months	• natural sunlight is readily available

- containers dry out quicker
- in-ground gardens and raised gardens don't dry out too quickly

- protected from the elements
- not protected from the elements

- potting soil is generally used, and no other fertilizer is required
- native soil needs to be amended, or fertile soil needs to be brought in

- less work involved in looking after the plants
- requires extensive labor to keep weeds away and the plants well-maintained

- less likely to be affected by pests
- more exposure to pests

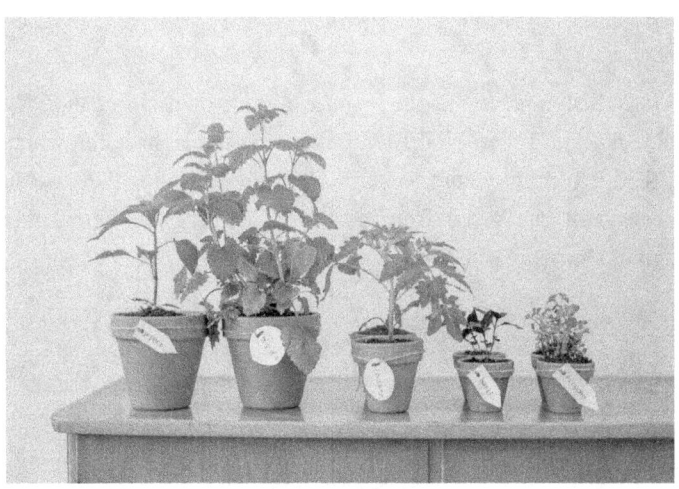

Growing plants indoors is easy but will require an investment in artificial lights to ensure the plants get the required sunlight —especially during winter.

Chapter 2
Choosing Your Herbs

Many different medicinal herbs can be grown either indoors or outdoors. It can be difficult choosing the right herbs when you don't know where to start. Here are a few of the easiest herbs you can grow from seeds or seedlings to help fight against an array of common ailments.

Name	• Peppermint (*Mentha piperita*)
Growing requirements	• Peppermint prefers full sunlight but can tolerate some shade.
	• Ideally grown in zones 3–8, but can grow in zones 9–10 when provided ample water and shade.
	• To promote high flavor, ensure the soil has a pH of 6.0–7.0.
Planting tips	• All mints are vicious spreaders and will take over a raised bed if not contained. It may be best to grow in a container.
	• Can be difficult to grow from seeds; get seedlings.
	• Plant 18–24 inches away from other plants.

Herbal Remedies & Natural Healing From Your Garden

Maintenance tips
- Peppermint will need 1–2 inches of water a week.
- Can tolerate moist soil but never soggy.

Health benefits
- Helps treat ailments such as stomach and digestive issues, blocked sinuses, motion or morning sickness, and headaches or migraines.
- A tea of peppermint can be cooled and used to soothe sunburn or enjoyed as is to promote sleep.

Warnings
- Excess ingestion of peppermint can lead to vomiting, heartburn, nausea, and dry mouth.
- Peppermint can interact with some medications.
  - It affects how quickly medicines are broken down by the liver, leading to changes in medicinal and side effects.

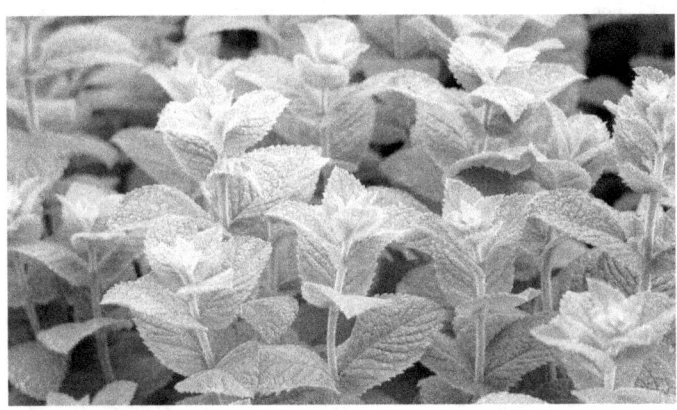

Name	• Oregano (*Origanum vulgare*)
Growing requirements	• Enjoys growing in full sun in zones 5–10, with a soil pH of 6.5–7.0.
Planting tips	• Oregano can be planted as seeds, cuttings, or seedlings. • Ensure they have 8–10 inches of space.
Maintenance tips	• This herb can be trimmed from the time it's 4 inches tall, allowing it to grow bushier. • It only requires an inch of water a week.
Health benefits	• Can be used to help ease coughs and fight back against infections, as it has antiviral, antibacterial, and antifungal properties. • A tea of oregano will also help calm nerves.
Warnings	• Consuming an excess of this herb will result in a possible upset stomach. • Oregano may have interactions with medications aimed at slowing blood clotting and lowering blood sugar.

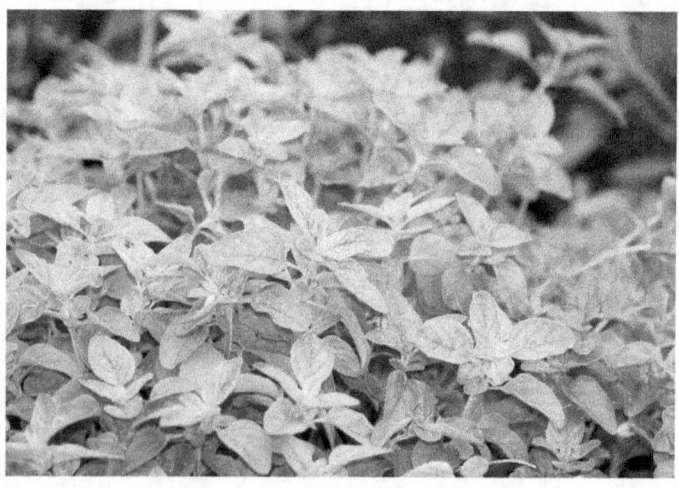

Herbal Remedies & Natural Healing From Your Garden

Name	• Calendula (*Calendula officinalis*)
Growing requirements	• Calendula prefers full sun but will tolerate some afternoon shade. • While this herb prefers zones 9–11, it can be grown from zones 2 upwards. • For the best results, plant in soil with a pH of 5.5–7.0.
Planting tips	• Individual plants should be separated by 6–18 inches. • Calendula can be grown from seeds or seedlings.
Maintenance tips	• To promote more flower production, clear away fading blooms (deadheading). • Calendula will need 1–1 ½ inches of water a week.
Health benefits	• The antifungal and antibacterial properties of calendula allow it to be useful in antibacterial creams as well as creams aimed at treating skin issues. It can also help to lower swelling in glands.
Warnings	• Calendula falls into the Asteraceae or Compositae (daisy) family and will cause allergies in anyone allergic to daisies, chrysanthemums, or marigolds. • This herb interacts with sedatives, making people sleepier than normal.

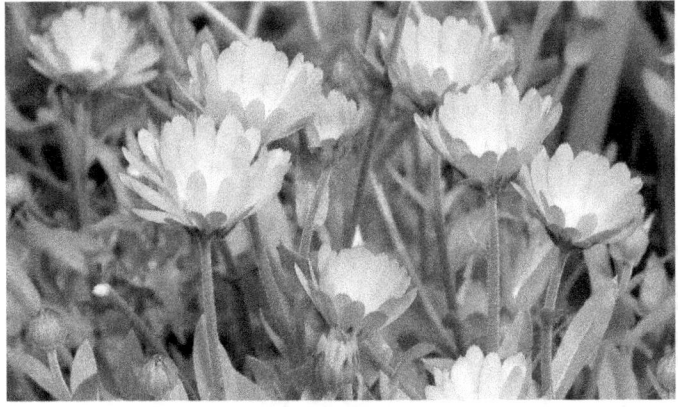

Name	• Tulsi, also known as holy basil (*Ocimum tenuiflorum*)
Growing requirements	• Tulsi prefers to grow in zones 10–11 but can grow comfortably in lower zones. It is frost-sensitive. • It's best to grow this herb in soil with a pH of 5–8 in a sunny location.
Planting tips	• Tulsi is grown from seeds, cuttings, or seedlings. • Plant at 12–18 inches away from other plants.
Maintenance tips	• Tulsi can be pruned once the plant has at least three sets of leaves on the stem. This will encourage more growth. • The plant will require an inch of water a week.
Health benefits	• This plant can be used to help improve energy and help manage stress.
Warnings	• Consuming too much tulsi will cause nausea or diarrhea. • This herb has interactions with medication to slow blood clotting or lower blood sugar. • Tulsi can also possibly cause a drop in thyroxine (thyroid hormone), causing an exacerbation of hypothyroidism.

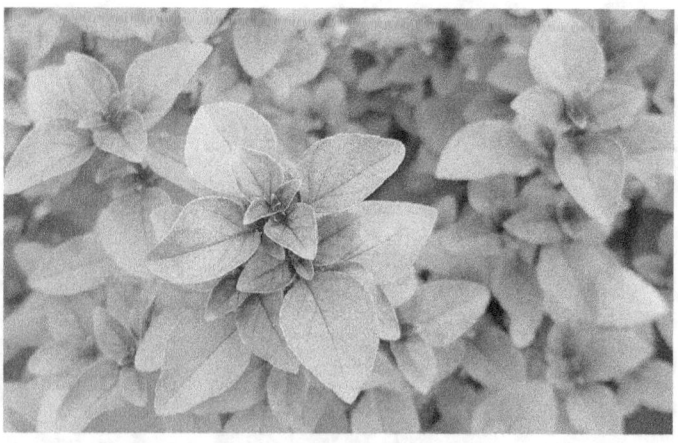

Herbal Remedies & Natural Healing From Your Garden

Name	• Echinacea, also known as coneflowers (*Echinacea purpurea*)
Growing requirements	• Echinacea enjoys early morning sun and some partial shade in the afternoon. • The soil should have a pH of 6.0–7.0. • Echinacea is comfortable growing in zones 3–9.
Planting tips	• This herb can be grown from seeds, though it may be best to get a seedling. • This is a drought-tolerant plant, so allow the soil to dry between waterings. • Plant this herb 12–15 inches from others.
Maintenance tips	• Deadheading will aid in more bloom production. • Will need about an inch of water a week.
Health benefits	• This plant is great for lowering the duration of colds and flu and may even help to boost the immune system.
Warnings	• Affects the liver's ability to break down some medications. • Avoid using it if you are suffering from autoimmune disorders, as it boosts immune function. • Avoid using if allergic to any flowers from the daisy family.

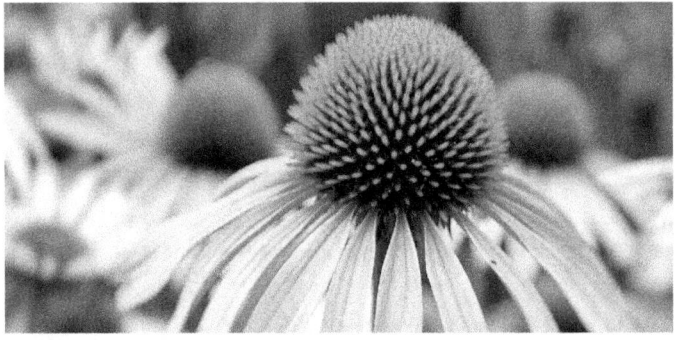

Olivia Phillips

Name	• Chamomile (*Matricaria chamomilla*, German chamomile)
Growing requirements	• Chamomile prefers full sun but will tolerate the shade. • Enjoys growing in zones 2–9 in a soil pH of 5.6–7.5.
Planting tips	• Grow this plant 8–11 inches away from others. • Can be grown in poor soils. • This herb is best grown from seedlings.
Maintenance tips	• It's important to trim chamomile to prevent it from becoming leggy. Deadheading will encourage more blooms. • This herb will need an inch of water a week when young. Once older, allow the soil to dry before watering again.
Health benefits	• This plant has a range of health benefits, from easing stomach pain and gas to promoting calmness and sleep, and can be made into a wash to treat conjunctivitis.
Warnings	• Those allergic to the daisy family should avoid this herb. • Chamomile may act similarly to estrogen, so avoid using it if going through hormone-sensitive conditions. • This herb may interact with anesthesia, so avoid taking it two weeks before surgery. • Chamomile also interacts with birth control and medications broken down by the liver, increases the effectiveness of sedatives, and can decrease the effectiveness of blood clotting medication.

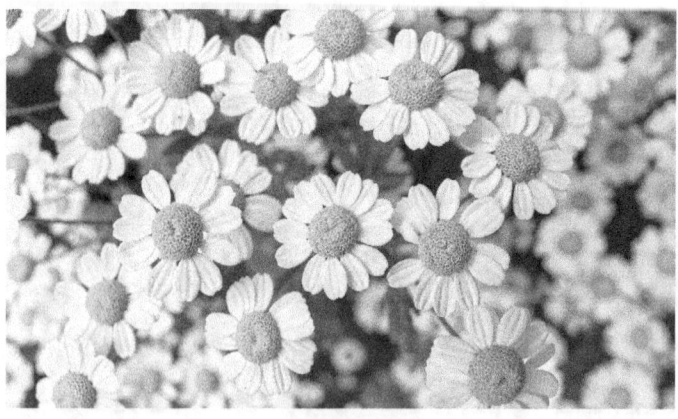

Please note that herbal remedies aren't recommended to anyone pregnant, breastfeeding, or under the age of two. Consult with a doctor before using a herbal remedy.

Part Two

Harvesting and Preparing Your Herbs

Now that your garden is producing an array of different herbs, it's time to discuss when to harvest and how to store the produce correctly. Once you have the prepared herbs, they can be used for many different remedies.

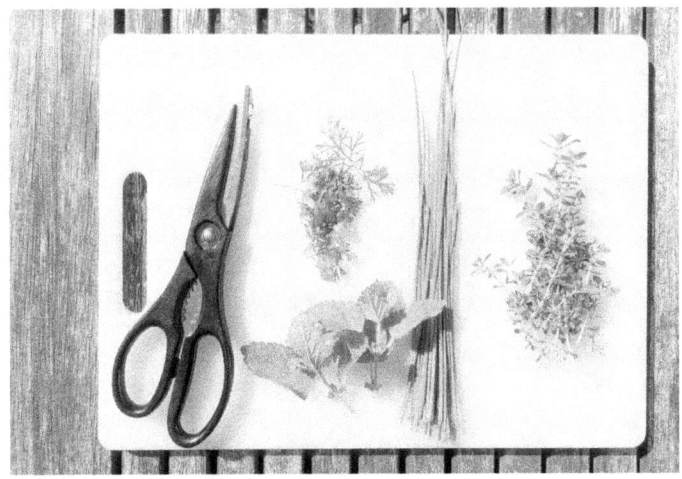

Chapter 3
Harvesting Techniques

Depending on the plant you're growing, there could be several parts that you could be harvesting. The most common part collected are the leaves, but the roots (ginger), bark (cinnamon), and flowers (calendula) are also harvestable.

Each part needs to be harvested at a specific time to allow them to maintain their medicinal properties for as long as possible. Annuals can be harvested in total before fall. However, perennials shouldn't be harvested later than late summer, allowing them enough time to recover before winter, which is especially important if they're growing outside.

Leaves can be harvested up until flowers start to be produced, which causes them to lose flavor. Never collect more than a third of the leaves at a time and no more than 75% of the total plant throughout the year. When harvesting leaves, ensure you cut between leaf nodules (between sets of leaves).

Flowers should be collected just after they open but before full bloom is reached. Cut the flower just below the green leaves (sepals or bracts) of the flower. If you want pods, allow the flowers to fade and collect the seed pods as they change from green to brown. Roots are best collected just before fall. The bark is best collected at the start of spring. Prune away excess branches and strip the outer bark to get the required inner bark.

When collecting leaves, flowers, buds, or fruit, ensure that it's done just as the dew starts to dry. As the temperatures rise, the volatile oils will evaporate, and the medicinal value of the harvest will be diminished. It's vital that you only harvest from plants that appear healthy.

Drying and Storing

While there are many ways to preserve your harvest, the most common and easiest is the drying method. When drying a large number of herbs, air drying is the best method to use.

1. Gently rinse any dust or dirt from the gathered material. Roots will need some scrubbing.
2. Spread the harvest on some paper towels and allow it to dry away from direct sunlight.
3. Strip the last two inches of leaves from stems before creating small bundles tied together with twine or rubber bands. Tie them tightly, as the stems will shrink as they dry.
4. Hang the bundles upside-down in a room, away from direct sunlight and heat. An empty room or cupboard with good airflow is perfect.
5. When seeds are being collected, hang the bundled harvest with a paper bag over it. Add a few punch

holes to allow airflow within the bag, but ensure that it's not near the bottom where the seeds would fall.

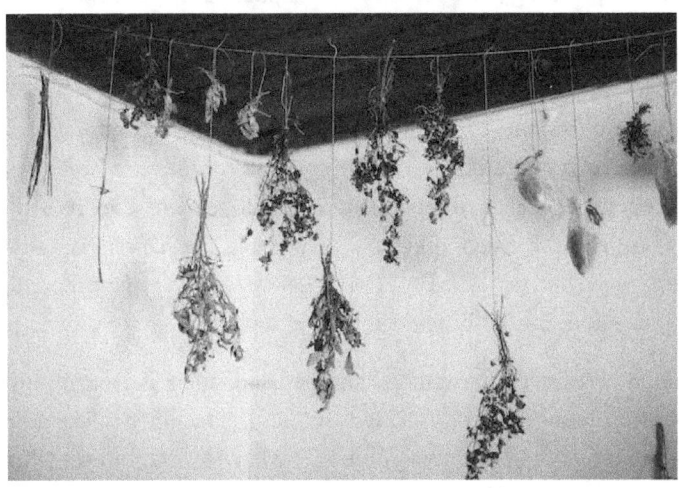

Instead of hanging herbs on a line, they can be placed on a screen and then added to a room under the same conditions as the bundled herbs. This method works well if you only want to dry leaves or roots. Roots will need to be sliced to ¼–½ an inch thick before drying.

Other alternatives to dry herbs include the use of an oven, dehydrator, or microwave, although these methods use a lot of electricity.

The harvest must be completely dry before storing, as this will prevent mold. Leaves should be brittle, while fruit, bark, and roots should snap when bent. Once fully dry, the harvest can be added to labeled airtight containers. Information that should be added to the label includes the common and Latin name of the plant, what part is preserved, and when it was preserved. Once this is complete, put the container in a cool, dry place that is away from direct sunlight. Ideally, separate containers according to how strong the scent is, as you don't want the strong scents to have an impact on the more delicate scents and flavors.

If living in a humid place, you may have to add a desiccator to the container. This can be done with packets of silica gel beads or some milk powder wrapped in a paper towel. These need to be checked now and again to ensure they're still working well. Even after you're sure that the harvest is fully dry, check it periodically. Dried harvests will remain potent for up to a year before needing to be replaced.

Other preservation methods can be used, such as freezing or storing in oil or alcohol. However, before deciding to use any of these methods, ensure you know what you want to do with your harvest, as how you preserve it will impact the recipe you want to use it in.

Seasonal Harvesting Guide

With so many plants that can be grown or foraged, it can be difficult to know when a plant will be ready to be harvested. Here is a quick harvesting guide of some herbs to remind you when certain plants can be harvested.

Spring and summer	• Leaves: basil, nettles, oregano, rosemary, and St. John's wort (flowers included)
	• Flowers: calendula (late spring), chamomile (late spring), and lavender (variant dependent)
	• Fruit: cayenne and other hot peppers (late summer)
Fall and winter	• Bulbs: garlic
	• Leaves: lemongrass
	• Fruit: rosehips
Extended	• Leaves: lemon balm (spring-fall), mints (late spring-early fall), sage (spring–winter), and winter savory (year-round)

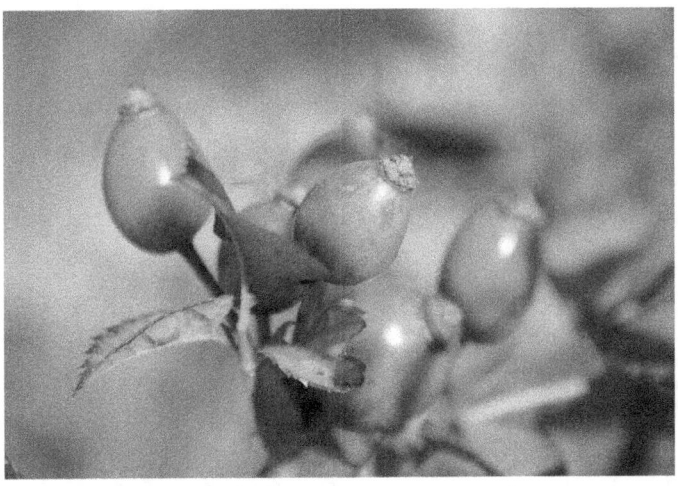

In the case of medicinal plants that have multiple parts that can be harvested, ensure that you harvest leaves before flowers appear, flowers before seed pods, and seed pods before they open and release seeds.

Chapter 4
Preparing Herbal Remedies

With your preserved medicinal plants, it's time to learn how to use them in various types of remedies. Herbal remedies can be prepared as teas, tinctures, salves, oil infusions, and more. Which you decide to make will depend on the ailment you're treating, but more on this later.

Tinctures

Tinctures are powerful liquid extracts that are made using high-proof alcohol or vinegar. Due to the strength, only a few drops under the tongue is all that's required. Tinctures can be made with fresh or dried ingredients, though the dried ingredients will make for a more potent tincture. To make a tincture:

1. Gather all the necessary ingredients and chop roughly.
2. Add everything to a jar that can seal.

3. Pour in the vinegar or high-proof alcohol to cover the ingredients. Dry ingredients need four times the volume of liquid, as they are more absorbent.

4. Seal the jar and allow it to soak for six weeks in a dark, cool place. Shake occasionally and top up as needed.

5. Strain the solids from the liquid.

6. Pour the liquids into clean, dark-colored, sealable containers, such as medicine dropper bottles.

7. Label well, stating if the tincture is made with fresh or dry ingredients, what liquid was used (vinegar or alcohol with its proof), the date made, and how the tincture should be used.

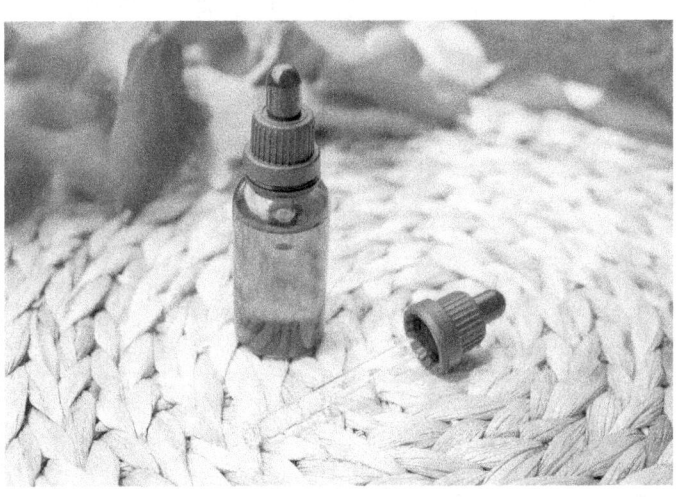

Teas

Teas are another liquid extract, although weaker, as the dried herbal components are allowed to soak in hot water before being drunk hot or cold. Fresh or dried components can be used. To make a tea:

1. Boil water, enough for a cup.
2. Select the components you want to steep, usually a blend. Add these to a tea strainer or ball.
3. Add the components to the boiled water. Use three times as much fresh as you would dry.
4. Pour the boiled water over the components and allow it to soak for 10–15 minutes before enjoying.

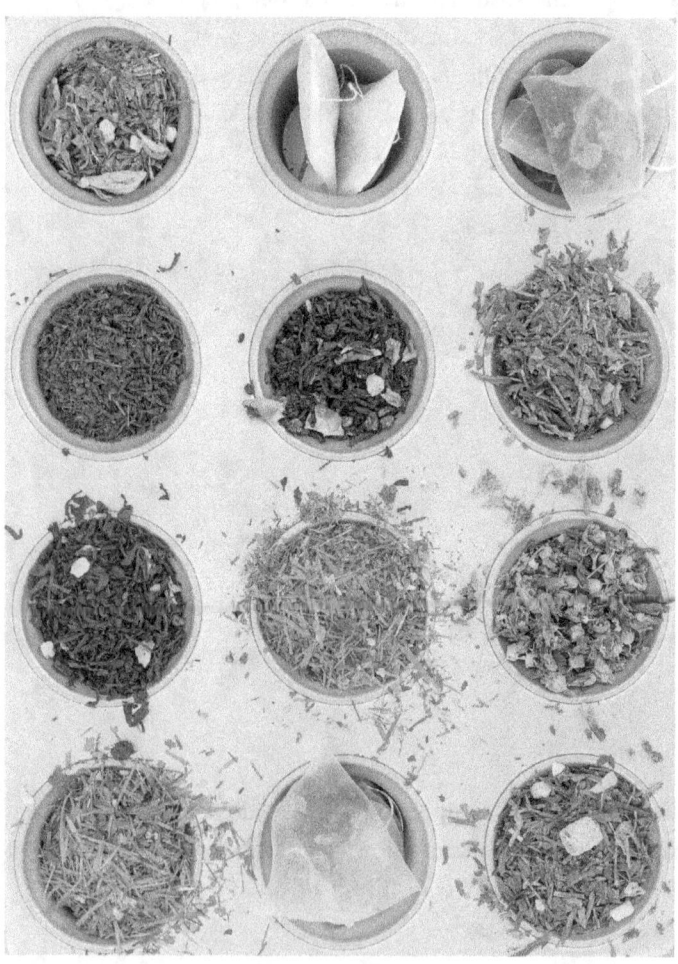

Oil Infusions

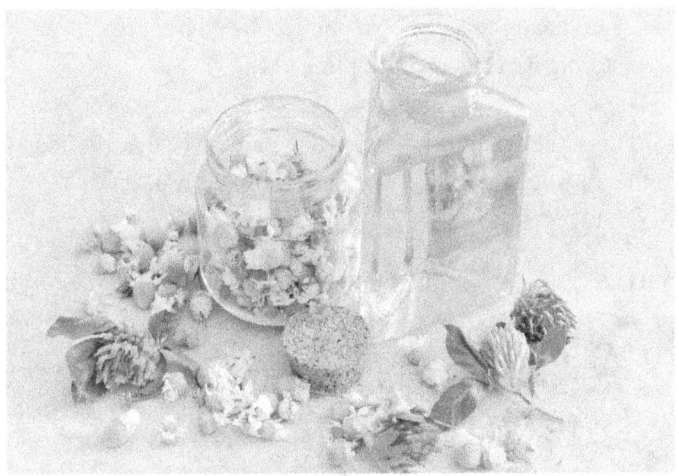

Oil infusions are similar to teas, but oil is used, and the steeping is significantly longer. Many carrier oils can be used, including coconut or olive oil. Oil infusions are needed if you want to make soaps, salves, creams, and even massage oils. It's a better idea to use dried ingredients when making an oil infusion. To make an oil infusion:

1. Add the dried components to a quart jar, leaving one to three inches headspace.
2. Pour the oil in, covering the material by at least an inch. The material will eventually surface, and the oil can be topped up.
3. Add a lid and shake.
4. Leave the jar on a sunny windowsill, covered with a brown paper bag, for two to three weeks. Shake daily. There may be some leakage, so place it onto some paper towels.

5. Strain all solids from the oil to prevent it from going rancid. Squeeze the solids to get all the oil out.
6. Add the oil to a clean jar and label well before storing it in a cool, dark place.

Adding some vitamin E—up to one percent of the solution—to the oil before storing will extend the shelf life.

Salves

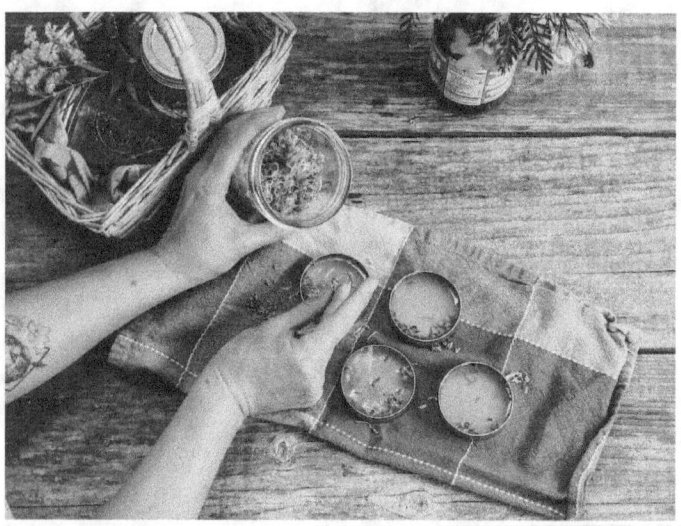

Salves are semi-solid creams made with beeswax or soy wax at room temperature. Before you can make a salve, an oil infusion or essential oils of the desired herb(s) are required. To make a salve:

1. Break the preferred wax into smaller pieces or get pellets.
2. Melt wax in a double boiler over a low temperature.

3. Pour the infused oil into the mixture and stir until well incorporated.
4. Remove from the heat, and add a few essential oil drops before pouring into clean tins or jars to cool.

The firmness of the salve is dependent on the wax. The more wax, the more firm; the less wax, the less firm. If a salve starts to harden as you pour it into the final container, reheat it over medium heat until liquid.

How to Create Herbal Remedies

In the beginning, it's best to stick to the recipes provided instead of creating unique remedies. Take the time to learn about the plants you're using and how they can affect people and interact with medication. Once you're more comfortable with various herbal remedies, then you can start experimenting.

- Keep a detailed notebook and take meticulous notes.
- Only experiment with plants that are safe for consumption.
- Start small and test rigorously through trial and error.
- Any plants used should be preserved and labeled well so you can refer back to them if something goes wrong with a batch.

Safety Guidelines

Herbal remedies aren't governed by the FDA, and few scientific studies have determined safety guidelines or recommended dosages for any homemade herbal remedies. Commercial herbal remedies come standard with dosage recommendations, and WebMD does have some recommendations for dosages when it comes to plant oils or other extracts. For example, when using peppermint oil, you can have 270–1,350 mg for up to 4 weeks, but there is no recommendation on how many dried leaves you can have (*Peppermint - Uses, Side Effects, and More*, n.d.).

When testing home remedies, keep an eye out for negative reactions that resemble allergies (hives, redness, itching), vomiting, nausea, headaches, dizziness, and even an upset stomach. These are usually signs that the dose may be too high. Consider talking to an herbalist, naturopathic doctor, or pharmacist to assist you in preventing high dosages and possible interactions.

Part Three

Herbal Remedies for Common Ailments

From burns to stomach issues to promoting sleep, this section contains a variety of recipes you can use to ease some common ailments.

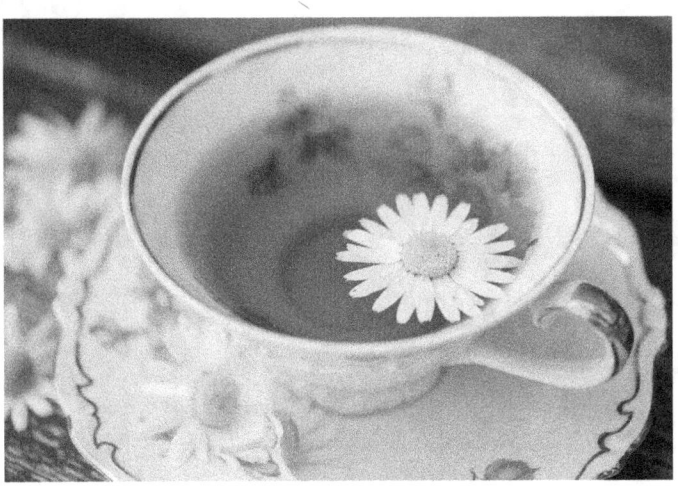

Chapter 5
Digestive Health

There is nothing worse than having an upset stomach. It leaves you too weak to function. Thankfully, there are a variety of herbs and spices that can help improve any digestive discomfort. Here are a few that will do wonders for your gut health.

Allspice *Pimenta dioica*	• promotes digestive enzymes and helps the gut to settle
	• avoid taking it together with blood clotting medicine
Caraway *Carum carvi*	• treats cramps, lower fermentation in the stomach, and eases nausea and gas in the bowels
	• when taken with peppermint, it may cause burping, heartburn, and nausea
	• may interact with diabetes medication, sedatives, and lithium
Chamomile *Matricaria chamomilla*	• eases flatulence, diarrhea, peptic ulcers, colic, gastritis, and gastrointestinal inflammation
	• may have interactions with many different medications
Cinnamon *Cinnamomum verum*	• improves appetite and fights *Helicobacter pylori* (bacteria that cause stomach ulcers) infections
	• can interfere with blood pressure and blood sugar medications

Dill *Anethum graveolens*	• lowers cramps and eases colic • seeds may cause menstruation or miscarriage • may interact with diabetes medication and lithium
Fennel *Foeniculum vulgare*	• improves digestive weakness, flatulence, cramping, and colic • avoid if suffering from gastroesophageal reflux or hormone-sensitive conditions
Gentian *Gentiana lutea*	• decreases stomachache, bloating, digestive weakness, and increases appetite • avoid taking with peptic ulcers or excess stomach acid
Ginger *Zingiber officinalis*	• eases bloating, digestive weakness, and nausea • avoid if suffering from stomach ulcers or on blood thinners
Globe artichoke *Cynora scolymus*	• eases constipation and bloating • avoid using it if there are gallbladder obstructions
Peppermint *Mentha piperita*	• often used to treat spasms and nausea • may cause dry mouth, nausea, vomiting, and heartburn
Marshmallow root *Althaea officinalis*	• helps treat gastroesophageal reflux, peptic ulcers, and gastritis • best avoided if on prescription drugs, speak to your doctor
Turmeric *Curcuma longa*	• often used to treat *H. pylori*, digestive weakness, peptic ulcers, and gastrointestinal inflammation • may affect blood thinning medication when used at high doses

Tea Recipes

Here's a collection of some soothing teas that will help get your digestion back on track.

Stomach Soothing Tea

Reach for this tea to help soothe an upset stomach. The peppermint will help lower the cramps, while the chamomile will soothe the pain.

Ingredients:

- ¼ oz dried orange peels
- ¼ oz fennel seeds
- ¼ oz dried ginger root
- 1 oz dried peppermint leaves
- 1 oz dried chamomile flowers

Directions:

1. In a dry mason jar, add all the ingredients and mix well.
2. Add 2–3 tablespoons of the mixture to a cup and pour in boiling water.
3. Allow to steep for 10 minutes.
4. Remove the solids and enjoy hot.

Digestive Aid Tea

Only a cup of this delicious tea is enough to settle an unhappy stomach.

Ingredients:

- ½ oz dried cinnamon
- ½ oz dried ginger
- 1 oz dried orange peel
- 1 oz dried licorice
- 3 ½ oz dried chamomile
- 3 ½ oz dried peppermint

Directions:

1. Blend all the ingredients in a mason jar.
2. Boil a quart of water.
3. Pour the hot water into a teapot or mason jar and add 8 teaspoons of the blend.
4. Steep for 15–20 minutes.
5. Remove solids and sweeten with some honey if needed.

Digestion Boosting Tea

If you're prone to digestive issues, add this tea to your daily meals to make the issues disappear. This blend is enough for a cup of soothing tea. If you have a lawn full of dandelions that haven't been poisoned, make them work for you. Dandelion helps support the liver during digestion.

Ingredients:

- ½ tsp roasted dandelion root
- ½ tsp dried cinnamon chips
- ½ tsp dried fennel seeds
- ½ tsp dried ginger
- 1 tsp dried chamomile flowers

Directions:

1. Add the ingredients to a tea strainer or ball before adding to the cup.
2. Add the boiling water and allow it to steep for 5–10 minutes.

Spasm Relieving Tea

Spasming guts hurt, so try some soothing lemon balm with peppermint. This combination will help soothe the cramps and pain associated with it.

Ingredients:

- ½ lemon slice, fresh
- 1 tsp dried fenugreek or fennel seeds (lightly crushed)
- 1 cinnamon stick
- 1 tsp dried lemon balm leaves
- 1 tsp dried peppermint leaves
- 3 cups water, boiled
- 1-inch fresh ginger, sliced (optional)
- 2 tsp honey (optional)
- 1-inch fresh turmeric, sliced (optional)

Directions:

1. Add all the ingredients, bar the optional ones, to a heat-safe pitcher.
2. Pour the boiled water over the ingredients.
3. Cover the pitcher and steep tea for 5–10 minutes.
4. Strain before adding any of the optional ingredients.
5. Enjoy with a garnish of mint leaves or a slice of orange or lemon.

Ayurvedic Digestion Tea

Also known as the CCF tea (cumin-coriander-fennel), this tea helps fight bloating, indigestion, and constipation while preventing gas and supporting digestion. To make a larger blend of this tea, fill a container with a third of each ingredient, then use less than a teaspoon per two cups of water.

Ingredients:

- ¼ tsp cumin seeds (less if you find it too strong)
- ¼ tsp coriander seeds
- ¼ tsp fennel seeds
- 2 cups of water

Directions:

1. Blend the ingredients into a large cup.
2. Boil the water and pour it over the ingredients, allowing them to steep for 4–5 minutes. Enjoy while hot.

If you don't have a blend prepared, no worries; several teas can be enjoyed to ease digestive discomfort. Try a cup of peppermint, oolong, Pu-erh (aged black tea), black tea, dandelion root, ginger, chamomile, licorice root, cardamom, or green tea.

Chapter 6
Cold and Flu Relief

There is nothing worse than being forced to stay in bed feeling miserable with a cold or flu. Luckily, there are some herbs and spices that can help lower the duration and severity of symptoms. With an array of preparations, you're surely to find something to help you feel better. Here are some of the plants you can use to get relief from colds and flu.

Astragalus *Astragalus membranaceus*	• helps strengthen and regulate the immune system, helping it to fight viral infections
	• can be used in capsules, tinctures, tablets, or teas
Black cumin *Nigella sativa*	• high in antioxidants, giving the immune system a boost
	• usually enjoyed in teas
Cinnamon *Cinnamomum verum*	• higher in antioxidants than most other herbal components, has anti-inflammatory, antifungal, and antibacterial properties
	• often used in foods and teas, but can be also used in tinctures

Echinacea *Echinacea purpurea*	• stimulates the immune system while easing cold and flu symptoms and lowering their duration • can be taken in tea, capsules, tinctures, or other extracts
Garlic *Allium sativum*	• stimulates the immune system and highly antimicrobial • generally used in food but can be used in extracts or capsules
Ginger *Zingiber officinale*	• anti-inflammatory, analgesic (pain-relief), and lowers severity and duration of illnesses • Used in food, extracts, teas, and capsules
Paprika *Capsicum annuum*	• high in vitamins A and C, which help to boost the immune system and reduce illness duration • can be consumed in many ways or added to salves
Peppermint *Mentha piperita*	• analgesic and anesthetic properties, and clears sinuses when inhaled • can be used in salves, teas, or oil infusions
Tulsi *Ocimum tenuiflorum*	• high in antioxidants and has germicide properties • can enjoy the leaves as is or dried in teas
Turmeric *Curcuma longa*	• reduces inflammation and is high in antioxidants • use a little black pepper to absorb better when consuming in teas or extracts

Illness Fighting Recipes

Illness can be fought by giving your immune system a much-needed boost! Here are a few different preparations to help you keep illness at the door.

Immune-Boosting Tincture

As soon as everyone around you starts to get sick, add a few drops of the immune-boosting tincture to your morning tea to give your immune system a wake-up call.

Ingredients:

- ½ oz dried chamomile
- 1 tsp dried ginger
- 1 tbsp honey
- 1 tsp cardamom seeds
- 1 oz dried astragalus root
- 1 cinnamon stick
- 1 oz dried angelica root
- 1 tsp dried orange peel
- 10 oz alcohol (100 proof vodka)

Directions:

1. Boil water and add 2 teaspoons to a mason jar with the honey. Stir until the honey is dissolved.
2. Allow the honey mixture to cool before adding the remaining ingredients, leaving the alcohol till last.
3. Seal and place in a cool, dark place for 2–4 weeks, shaking daily. The longer it's stored, the stronger it'll become.
4. Strain the solids through a cheesecloth and store the tincture in a dark, airtight container away from direct sunlight.

Elderberry Syrup

Elderberries are high in vitamin C, which boosts the immune system. If you are already sick, this syrup will reduce excess mucus and ease sore throats.

Ingredients:

- ¾ cup dried elderberries
- 1 tsp ground ginger
- 1 cup honey
- 1 cinnamon stick
- 3 cups water
- 4 whole cloves

Directions:

1. Add all the ingredients, bar the honey, to a saucepan, then bring to a boil.
2. Once a boil is achieved, lower the temperature until the mixture starts to simmer. Simmer for 30 minutes.
3. Remove from heat and pour the mixture through a strainer lined with cheesecloth into a clean jar. Squeeze the cheesecloth lightly to ensure all the liquid is strained out.
4. While the liquid is still warm (not hot), dissolve the honey.
5. Allow the mixture to cool completely before adding a lid to the jar and placing it in the fridge.
6. Enjoy up to a tablespoon a day as is, or mix it with other drinks.

Chest-Clearing Rub

A chest rub is one of the best ways to clean any nasal blockages and offer some instant relief while fighting colds and flu.

Ingredients:

- ½ cup coconut oil
- ¼ cup grated beeswax or soy wax
- ¼ cup olive oil
- 20 drops of eucalyptus essential oil
- 20 drops of cedarwood or peppermint essential oil

Directions:

1. Add the two oils and wax to a clean jar.
2. Add 2 inches of water to a saucepan and heat it over low heat.
3. Place the jar in the saucepan; it will act as a double boiler.
4. Stir the oils and wax until melted and well combined. Use a wooden spoon.
5. Once well mixed, remove the jar from the saucepan and allow it to cool for a few minutes before stirring in the essential oils.
6. Pour the salve into a prepared tin or jar and allow it to cool to a solid state.

Immune Supporting Tea

If you start to feel a tickle in the back of your throat, enjoy a cup of immune-supporting tea to give the immune system a much-needed boost.

Ingredients:

- ¼ cup echinacea
- ¼ cup dried elderberries

- ¼ cup rose hips
- ¼ cup chamomile flowers
- ¼ cup astragalus
- 1 tsp honey (optional)

Directions:

1. In a large jar, add all the dried ingredients and mix well.
2. Place 2–3 teaspoons of the blend in a cup or strainer before pouring in boiled water.
3. Allow the mixture to steep for 10 minutes before removing solids.
4. Sweeten as desired.

Chapter 7
Skin Care Solutions

Minor burns, cuts, abrasions, and rashes are hardly anything that requires an emergency room visit. However, these injuries are a pain to have to deal with and can linger longer than we want. Instead of going to your closest pharmacy to deal with slight injuries, reach for the following botanicals to alleviate pain and itching.

Aloe *Aloe vera*	• the gel within the leaves can be applied directly to minor burns and wounds to assist in healing
Calendula *Calendula officinalis*	• supports the regeneration of tissues, aiding healing • anti-inflammatory and has a calming effect
Chamomile *Matricaria chamomilla*	• anti-inflammatory properties that assist in relieving itching, swelling, and redness
Comfrey *Symphyum officinale*	• anti-inflammatory and regenerative • helps treat burns, eczema, and minor cuts
Dandelion *Taraxacum officinale*	• a gentle botanical that helps alleviate eczema and other skin issues

Lavender *Lavandula augustiflora*	• anti-inflammatory, antibacterial, antifungal, and full of antioxidants
	• soothes itching from bug bites and stings and offers pain relief from burns
Peppermint *Mentha piperita*	• soothes itchy skin
Plantain *Plantago ovata* *P. lanceolata*	• generally macerated and applied to stings as a poultice to soothe
Tea tree *Melaleuca alternifolia*	• soothes itching from rashes and insect bites
Turmeric *Curcuma longa*	• soothes pain from cuts, abrasions, and other lesions

While some plants are considered weeds, know that these plants were used for centuries by ancient humans before today's botanicals were grown for specific purposes.

Skin Soothing Recipes

Before trying any of the salves in the recipe section, it's important to do an allergy test. Apply a little salve to the inside of the arm or elbow crook and wait a few minutes to see if there's a reaction. Discontinue use if there is any adverse reaction.

Aloe and Lavender Burn Salve

From sunburn to minor heat burns, this salve will not only soothe the pain but improve healing and lower the chance of scarring. Remember to cool a heat burn with water before applying salve.

Ingredients:

- ½ cup coconut oil
- 1 tsp vitamin E oil
- 2 tbsp aloe vera gel
- 2 tbsp beeswax or soy wax
- 15 drops of lavender essential oil

Directions:

1. In a double boiler, melt the wax and oil and stir until combined.
2. Remove mixture from heat and pour into a prepared tin.
3. Allow to cool for a few minutes before stirring in the remaining ingredients.
4. Allow to fully cool, label, and store.

Bug Bite Soothing Salve

Mosquitoes are a pain during the summer, but they don't have to be with this calendula-infused salve. It can even help heal minor cuts and skin irritations, such as razor burns.

Ingredients for Calendula-infused Oil:

- ¾ cup olive oil, sweet almond, or jojoba oil
- ½ cup dried calendula flowers

Ingredients for Salve:

- ½ oz chopped beeswax
- ¾ cup olive oil, jojoba oil, or sweet almond

- 4 oz calendula-infused oil
- 20 drops of lavender essential oil (optional)

Directions for Infused Oil:

1. Add the flowers to fill ¾ of a mason jar before adding the oil to cover them.
2. Seal and allow the mixture to seep for 4–6 weeks away from direct sunlight.
3. Strain the mixture through cheesecloth and store the oil away, well labeled, and in a dark, cool place.

Directions for Salve:

1. Add the beeswax and oil to a double boiler and heat until the wax melts. Stir to mix well.
2. Remove the mixture from heat, allowing it to cool slightly before adding the essential oils.
3. Pour the mixture into the prepared container and allow to fully cool before sealing.
4. Label and store in a cool, dry place.

Lavender Skin Soother

Whether minor burns, rashes, or other skin irritations, this soothing lavender salve not only repairs damaged skin but also helps soothe nerves. A thin film of salve is enough, so don't overdo it.

Ingredients:

- 1 cup lavender-infused oil
- 4 tbsp (~ 1 oz) beeswax pastilles (pellets)

- 20-25 drops of lavender essential oil
- 4-5 drops of other essential oils of choice (chamomile, ylang-ylang, rosemary, etc., optional)

Directions:

1. To a double boiler, add the lavender-infused oil and the beeswax.
2. Over low heat, melt the wax while stirring until everything is well incorporated.
3. Remove from the heat and add the essential oils once the mixture has cooled a little.
4. Pour the mixture into prepared containers.
5. Allow the mixture to solidify at room temperature before adding the lids.
6. Label and store in a cool, dry area.

Herbal Burn Salve

To make this salve, you'll need several premade-infused oils.

Ingredients:

- ½ tsp sea buckthorn oil
- ½ tsp calendula-infused olive oil
- 1 tsp burdock leaf-infused oil
- 1 tsp comfrey-infused olive oil
- 1 ¼ tsp beeswax
- 1 ½ tsp St. John's wort-infused olive oil

Directions:

1. Add all the ingredients to a double boiler and heat over low temperature until the wax melts.
2. Mix well and remove from heat until everything is well incorporated.
3. Pour into prepared tin or jar and allow to fully cool before adding their lids.
4. Ensure the containers are well labeled before storing them away.

Chapter 8
Stress and Sleep

Everyone is constantly busy trying to survive, so much so that they don't have time to deal with the stress they're under. Constant stress can lead to anxiety, depression, and poor sleep. To help alleviate some of the symptoms associated with stress and poor sleep, here are some botanicals that may soothe anxiety and deal with insomnia.

Ashwagandha
Withania somnifera
- helps lower symptoms associated with depression, fight fatigue, and lowers stress and anxiety
- Promotes concentration and mental focus while easing insomnia and promoting sleep

Chamomile
Matricaria recutita
- lowers nervousness and anxiety, promoting relaxation and making it easier to fall asleep

English Lavender
Lavandula angustifolia
- helps lower anxiety and cortisol (stress hormone), eases depression, and improves relaxation, therefore aiding sleep

Passionflower
Passiflora incarnata
- lowers anxiety, depression, and nervousness, eases insomnia, and promotes relaxation

Peppermint *Mentha piperita*	• relaxes muscles, easing tension, allowing sleep to be better • has some sedative effects
St. John's Wort *Hypericum perforatum*	• boosts the production of serotonin, which in turn helps lower symptoms of depression and easing sleep
Tulsi *Ocimum tenuiflorum*	• settles cortisol and fights back against depression and anxiety
Valerian root *Valeriana officinalis*	• helps lower anxiety and insomnia and relieves stress • consume in moderation as it can cause headaches and dizziness

Lemon balm also has a calming effect, plus it tastes great in tea and can make up for some of the more bitter botanicals.

Recipes to Soothe Stress and Promote Sleep

Enjoy some tasty herbal remedies to help you unwind from the day and promote healthy sleeping habits.

Calming Tea

The rich red color of this tea is from the hibiscus. Hibiscus is high in antioxidants that help fight stress. This recipe allows you to make as much or as little of the blend as you want.

Ingredients:

- 1 part chamomile
- 1 part lavender blossoms
- 2 parts passion flower
- 2 parts hibiscus flowers

- 2 parts lemon balm

Directions:

1. Mix the quantity of herbs you want and seal in a glass jar until ready to use.
2. When ready to enjoy a cup of tea, boil water and add a teaspoon of the blend to a tea strainer.
3. Pour the boiling water over the blend and allow it to steep for 5–7 minutes before enjoying.

Sleepytime Tea

Sleepytime tea helps ease insomnia through its calming and relaxing properties from a variety of anxiety-busting botanicals.

Ingredients:

- ¼ oz chamomile
- ¼ oz lemon balm
- ¼ oz rosebuds or petals
- ¼ oz passionflower

Directions:

1. To a bowl, add all the ingredients and mix well before storing.
2. Add a large teaspoon of the blend to a cup of boiled water, allowing it to steep for at least 5 minutes before enjoying.

Anti-Anxiety Tincture

To prevent anxiety from becoming chronic, take a few drops under the tongue to help when you start to feel a little overwhelmed.

Ingredients:

- 0.5 oz cinnamon
- 0.5 oz chamomile flowers
- 0.5 oz holy basil
- 0.5 oz lemon balm
- 100 proof vodka (50% alcohol)

Directions:

1. Add all the dried ingredients to a mason jar before pouring the alcohol over it.
2. Seal well and place in a dark spot for six weeks, shaking daily.
3. Strain the solids from the liquids using a cheesecloth. Continue to strain until no solids remain in the liquid.
4. Pour the liquid into a sealable, dark container and store it away from direct sunlight. Ensure the bottle is well labeled.

Sweet Dreams Tea

The sweet dreams tea uses a combination of fresh and dried ingredients. However, if you don't have access to fresh ingredients, the dried variety can be used.

Ingredients:

- 1 tbsp fresh mint
- 1 tbsp lemon balm
- 1 tbsp fresh or dried lavender buds
- 2 tbsp fresh or dried chamomile buds
- 8 fresh rose petals

Directions:

1. Add all the ingredients to a tea strainer or French press.
2. Pour 2–3 boiled water over the dried ingredients.
3. Allow to steep for 12 minutes before removing the tea strainer or pressing down the French press and pouring off the liquid to serve.

Part Four
Building Your Home Apothecary

Now that you're more comfortable growing, harvesting, and using botanicals in a range of remedies, it's time to build up a private apothecary. In the next section, we'll discuss how to organize your apothecary—along with the necessary tools and other ingredients—as well as look at how to personalize remedies for specific needs and other complex remedy preparations.

Chapter 9
Assembling Your Herbal Toolkit

When creating a home apothecary, there are vital tools that will make the journey easier. What your apothecary will need is up to you, as well as what remedies you'll be preparing. What you need should be broken down into herbs and tools required.

When deciding on what herbs you want, divide them into six groups:

- Adaptogens that help manage stress; astragalus, turmeric, tulsi, and skullcap
- Immune modulators that help support immunity; astragalus, ginger, elderberry, and tulsi
- Carminatives that help with soothing upset digestive systems; chamomile, peppermint, ginger, and skullcap
- Anti-inflammatories that lower inflammation and help with pain; calendula, chamomile, nettle, yarrow, turmeric, and slippery elm

- Antimicrobial herbs to help fight infections from bacteria, viruses, and fungi; garlic, calendula, peppermint, yarrow, turmeric, and echinacea
- Nutritive herbs that aid in general well-being; garlic, dandelion root, and elderberry

If your garden doesn't support the mass production of botanicals required for your remedies, purchase them from reputable sources.

When it comes to tools and other ingredients, you're spoiled for choice, depending on the types of preparations that are made.

Kitchen tools	• kettle, pots, double boiler, tea strainer, cheesecloth, mixing bowls, scale, measuring tools, motor and pestle (making powers), and funnel
Garden tools	• sharp scissors, sheers, and knives for harvesting
Containers	• sealable glass containers, amber bottles (for tinctures, with lids or droppers), and tins
Solvents	• alcohol (quality and high proof), honey, glycerin, vinegar, distilled water, and carrier oils (olive, sweet almond, or coconut)
Waxes and butters	• beeswax, soy wax, carnauba wax, or candelilla wax • shea, cocoa, kokum, or avocado butter
Extra scents	• quality essential oils
Miscellaneous	• labels and notebooks (one per preparation or divided into chapters)

As you gain more confidence in creating an apothecary, you'll find other tools to make the preparations easier.

Organizing the Apothecary

How your apothecary is organized is dependent on the amount of space you have. A smaller apothecary is easier to maintain, while a larger one will require more work and planning in the long run.

First and foremost, the apothecary is there to store the remedies to keep their potency for as long as possible. When remedies are stored correctly, they will retain their potency for longer. An apothecary doesn't need to be a dust cabinet secluded somewhere in your home. It's a living documentation of your journey to creating herbal remedies.

The best way to start an apothecary is to divide your various ingredients and preparations into groups. Not only will this identify what you have available, but it will make it easier to keep track of everything. Start by dividing everything into:

- fresh
- dried
- tinctures
- salves
- oil infusions
- essential oils

Once grouped, you can assign each group a duration to remain potent. Fresh herbs will last up to a week in the fridge, while dried herbs in an airtight container will last one to two years. It's best to keep dried herbs intact, as powdered herbs will only last six months to a year. Tinctures made with alcohol will last two to five years, while quality essential oils will last up to 8 years. However, this is dependent on the type of essential oils, as some citrus essential oils usually only remain potent for up to two years. Salves, when stored correctly, can last from six months to three years. Knowing the shelf life of your preparations will give you an indication of how often you should be rotating old stock out for new stock.

Each item should be labeled well with the name of the herb or a list of ingredients along with the preparation. This should be followed by the date when the ingredients were stored away or made. It's also a good idea to list the purpose of the preparation.

Once a label is added, it's time to store the containers. Generally, to maintain the potency of the preparation, the container should be kept in a cool and dry location, away from direct sunlight. Ideally, the storage area should be tiered so it's easier to see the containers. Something like a cabinet, bookcase, or cupboard is ideal. You can even hang a dust sheet over the front to prevent excess sunlight from getting to the remedies.

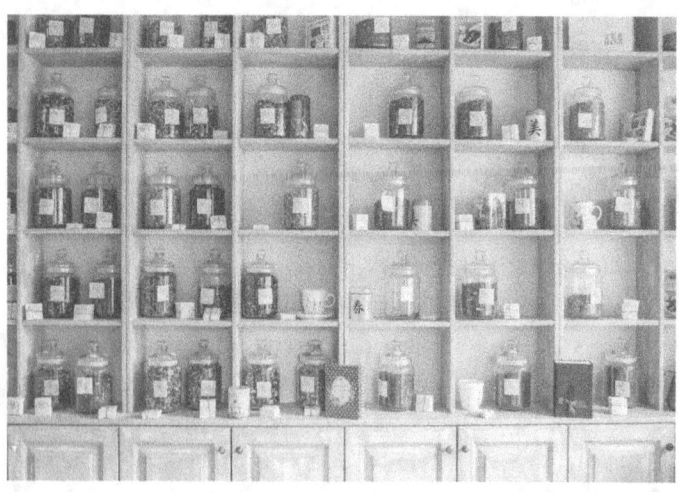

Wherever you decide to store your remedies, ensure they're in a place of convenience and can easily be checked. You can even draw a plan in your notebook describing where certain remedies will be placed. Develop a system that best suits your needs.

Chapter 10
Advanced Herbal Preparations

If you feel you're ready to continue your herbal remedy adventure, here are a few more types of preparations you can try your hand at.

Hydrosols

Hydrosols, also known as distillates, are created when essential oils are distilled from fresh plant material. They are the water-soluble parts, while the essential oils are the oil-soluble parts. The hydrosols have similar properties to the essential oils (calming, relaxing, or stress relief) but are considered gentler on the skin, as essential oils need to be in a carrier oil to be as gentle. These liquids are faintly scented and can be used in perfumes, skin toners, food flavorings, and alternative medicine. The best-known hydrosol is rose water.

Hydrosols only last three to six months in the fridge, so it's a good idea to make these when you need them instead of storing them. Making a hydrosol is simple but requires several tools to make it so.

Making a Hydrosol

Pick the botanical(s) you wish to use, only using fresh, as you're after the water-soluble parts. You'll need several cups worth. Then, you'll need a large pot, large enough to fit a large bowl, a smaller bowl, and the pot's inverted lid. Lastly, you'll need a stove, water, and ice.

1. Place the pot on the stove and add the large bowl upside down and the smaller bowl resting on the larger right side up.
2. Pack the botanicals around the larger bowl before covering them with water.
3. Heat the water until it's boiling, then lower the heat to bring it to a simmer.
4. Place the pot lid upside down so the handle is over the smaller bowl. Fill the top of the inverted pot lid with ice.
5. Allow the pot to simmer for 30 minutes, letting the steam condense against the ice-cold pot lid.
6. Replace the ice as needed.
7. After 30 minutes, remove the pot from the heat and allow it to cool.
8. Once cool, remove the lid, and you'll note the collected liquid in the smaller bowl. This will be a mixture of the hydrosol and some essential oils.
9. Scoop the essential oils off if you don't want them, decant the liquid into a dark container, and place in the fridge until you're ready to use them.

Extracts

Several extracts have already been discussed (tinctures and teas), but there are several other extract preparations that don't include water or alcohol. Different types of solvents will result in different kinds of extracts and have an impact on what is extracted from the plant.

Water extracts result in infusions and decorations. Teas are a type of infusion, as water is added to the botanicals and then allowed to steep to extract the benefits. Decoctions are when the botanicals are boiled in the water to make a more concentrated form of infusion.

Alcohol extractions result in tinctures, and while not popular, tinctures can also be extracted with vinegar. Apple cider vinegar is a particular favorite because of its array of health benefits. However, if you'd prefer to have an alcohol-free extraction, try glycerin as an extraction solvent. Glycerin also brings a natural sweetness that will help with the bitterness of these types of extractions. Other extracts you can consider are the oil infusions and, if you have it on hand, honey or syrup infusions.

These final extracts take significantly longer than decoctions and infusions, as the materials (usually dry) will need to soak in the solvent for three to four weeks with daily shakes. What better way to sweeten your herbal teas than with honey that is infused with the goodness of your preferred herbs?

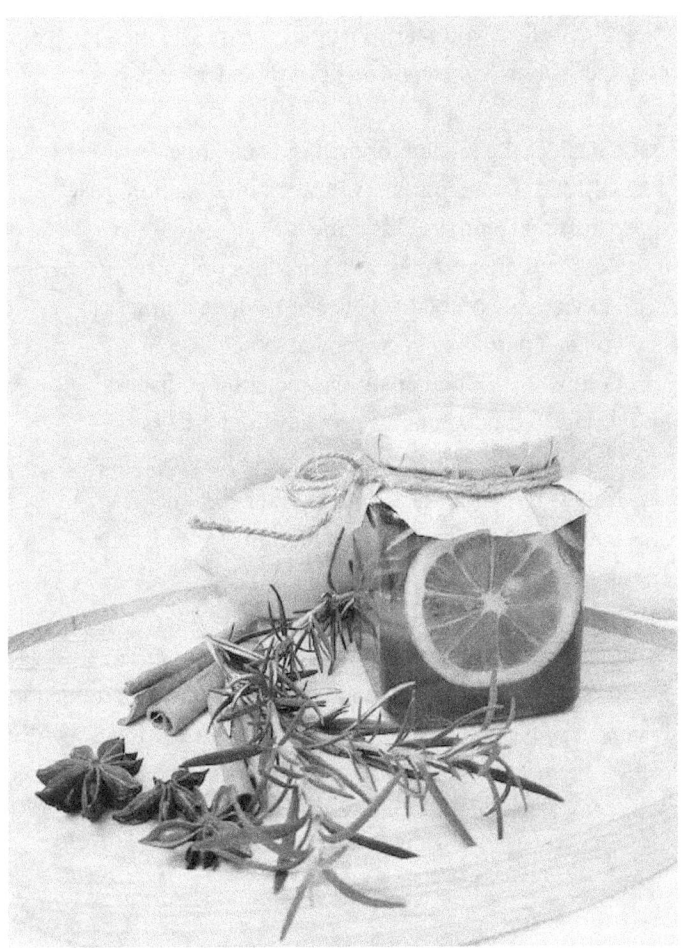

Personalizing Remedies

You may be feeling more confident in trying new concoctions. While there are many recipes you can try online, these recipes may not be what you're looking for. If there is a particular ailment you want to treat or you want to switch out ingredients due to an allergy, you will need to do some research. Before you start changing recipes or making your own, there are a few steps you need to understand.

- Consider the ailment or the needs that must be fulfilled (boost immunity, lower inflammation, ease pain, and so on) by this remedy.
- Research the botanicals that are generally used to alleviate the problem. This can be done online, or you can purchase a few reputable books.
- Follow up with other similar recipes and discuss dosage with doctors, naturopaths, or herbalists.
- Consider possible interactions and allergies.
- Make meticulous notes while you experiment. Write down the tastes, colors, and effectiveness of your homebrewed remedies.

It's important to remember that you aren't qualified to diagnose or suggest treatments to anyone, as you are not trained to do so. Always show your notes to a professional before testing them on yourself to avoid interactions with other medications and supplements you may be on.

Conclusion

Modern society is too quick to reach for over-the-counter medication or rush to an emergency room with common ailments. Common ailments can easily be treated at home if you know enough about different botanicals.

Herbal remedies have been around since the first ancient humans started exploring the environment around them and seeing how they could benefit them. These remedies have stood the test of time; they were first passed down verbally before being transcribed and are now considered common knowledge to some.

Many of these herbal remedies can be grown in your own backyard or indoors if you have no space outside. Many of these herbs make for great companion plants in vegetable gardens, as well as tasty additions to meals. However, they are best saved to create an array of different herbal remedies that can be used for daily ailments.

Whether you're feeling down and need a pick-me-up or are struggling to fall asleep, there are many herbs that you can

Conclusion

use to help ease you into a happier existence. The most important part of using herbal remedies is understanding that these are not cure-alls and aren't as stringently tested by the FDA as pharmaceutical drugs are. This means the doses of herbal remedies aren't as well-researched as those of pharmaceutical drugs.

This is not to say that herbal remedies don't have a place in treating common ailments. After all, pharmaceutical drugs originated from the botanical remedies of the past.

When choosing to treat common ailments with herbal remedies, it's vital to do your research on what possible interactions and allergies may be present. Once you know what herbs are safe to use, you can further your research into what properties these herbs have.

Peppermint is great for settling an upset stomach, but too much can cause heartburn. There is a delicate balance that must be observed when using herbal remedies. However, once you have achieved this, there are many different remedies and preparations you can make and store for future use.

Creating an apothecary will not only help you have an organized space where you can display your craft but also give you ready access to what you need when needed. That said, different preparations will require different methods of creation and storage. Try a few simple recipes with simple preparations for common ailments before moving on to those that are more complex.

Once you have the prepared remedies, be sure to come back and check on the quality, as some preparations can last longer than others. Leaving a remedy past its prime will result in a lower potency, not allowing it to fulfill its intended purpose.

Conclusion

Creating unique remedies can be a fun way to deal with problems you wouldn't want to bother a doctor with, but it's not there to replace your doctor. Your herbal garden can revitalize your soul and body, but the herbal remedies within this book are but a taste of a wider world of herbalism. Never stop learning and keep trying new recipes, enjoying the benefits you get from remaining healthy without needlessly resorting to pharmaceutical drugs.

Start your herbal garden today to benefit from not only being out in nature but also creating unique remedies and pick-me-up preparations that will bring an array of benefits to your life. Nothing is stopping you, so get started!

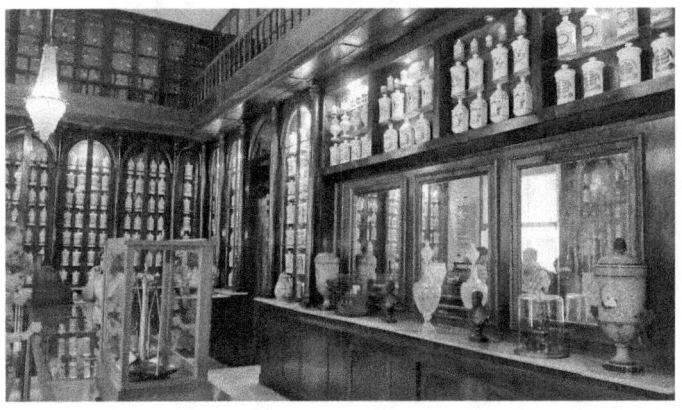

References

Aayushi, G. (2021, April 19). *These 7 stress-relief herbs will also work against your anxiety*. Healthshots. https://www.healthshots.-com/mind/mental-health/these-7-stress-relief-herbs-will-also-work-against-your-anxiety/

Adamant, A. (2021, December 23). *How to grow tulsi (indoors or outside)*. Practical Self Reliance. https://practicalselfreliance.com/how-to-grow-tulsi/

Allspice - Uses, side effects, and more. (n.d.). WebMD. https://www.webmd.-com/vitamins/ai/ingredientmono-81/allspice

Amy. (2021, March 14). *How to decide where to put your garden*. Gardens That Matter. https://gardensthatmatter.com/choose-garden-location/

Arora, D. (2023, June 22). 9 immunity boosting herbs to beat COVID-19! *PharmEasy Blog*. https://pharmeasy.in/blog/9-immunity-boosting-herbs-to-beat-covid-19/

Ask an herbalist: What is an herbal extract? (2022, February 2). *Herb Pharm*. https://www.herb-pharm.com/blogs/ask-an-herbalist/ask-an-herbalist-what-is-an-herbal-extract

Axe, J. (2022, February 1). *Homemade vapor rub*. Dr. Axe. https://draxe.-com/beauty/homemade-vapor-rub/

Bedosky, L. (2022, December 1). *7 herbs and spices that may help boost immunity naturally*. Everyday Health. https://www.everydayhealth.-com/diet-nutrition/herbs-and-spices-that-may-help-boost-immunity-naturally/

Boeckmann, C. (2023a, July 10). *Oregano*. Old Farmer's Almanac. https://www.almanac.com/plant/oregano

Boeckmann, C. (2023b, August 14). *Coneflowers*. The Old Farmer's Almanac. https://www.almanac.com/plant/coneflowers

Boyles, M. (2023, October 13). *12 uses for mint leaves, from health to home*. The Old Farmer's Almanac. https://www.almanac.com/12-uses-mint-leaves-health-home

Brief History Herbal Medicine. (2018, August 10). Herbal Clinic - Swansea. https://www.herbalclinic-swansea.co.uk/herbal-medicine/a-brief-history-of-herbal-medicine/

Burgess, L. (n.d.). 7 herbs to support digestive concerns. *Endeavour*.

References

https://www.endeavour.edu.au/about-us/blog/7-herbs-support-digestive-concerns/

Calendula - Uses, side effects, and more. (n.d.). WebMD. https://www.web-md.com/vitamins/ai/ingredientmono-235/calendula

Candice. (2022, May 28). *5 benefits of growing your own herbs.* My Little Green Garden. https://mylittlegreengarden.com/5-benefits-of-growing-your-own-herbs/

Caraway - Uses, side effects, and more. (n.d.). WebMD. https://www.web-md.com/vitamins/ai/ingredientmono-204/caraway

Ceylon cinnamon - Uses, side effects, and more. (n.d.). WebMD. https://www.webmd.com/vitamins/ai/ingredientmono-330/ceylon-cinnamon

Christelle. (2020, June 10). *How to make a tincture for anxiety.* Perma-crafters. https://www.permacrafters.com/how-to-make-a-tincture-for-anxiety/

Cummings, G. (2017, September 1). *10 common digestive herbs and their health benefits.* Evening Standard. https://www.standard.co.uk/going-out/foodanddrink/10-common-digestive-herbs-and-how-they-benefit-your-health-a3624266.html

DeannaCat. (2023, August 28). *How to make homemade lavender salve to soothe skin & nerves.* Homestead and Chill. https://homesteadandchill.-com/how-to-make-lavender-salve/

Dill - Uses, side effects, and more. (n.d.). WebMD. https://www.webmd.-com/vitamins/ai/ingredientmono-463/dill

Echinacea - Uses, side effects, and more. (n.d.). WebMD. https://www.web-md.com/vitamins/ai/ingredientmono-981/echinacea

Essential Wholesale and Labs. (2022, February 21). Extracts, distillates, hydrosols, and tinctures – What are they and what's the difference? https://blog.essentialwholesale.com/extracts-distillates-hydrosols-tinctures/

Evans, E., & Davis, I (2019, November 11). *Harvesting and Preserving Herbs for the Home Gardener | NC State Extension Publications.* NC State Extension. https://content.ces.ncsu.edu/harvesting-and-preserving-herbs-for-the-home-gardener

Fletcher, J. (2023, March 3). *What is an herbal tincture? Recipes and uses.* Medical News Today. https://www.medicalnewstoday.com/arti-cles/324149

Gardiner, B. (2023, November 8). *Start an amazing home apothecary with these 22 must-have herbs and tools.* The Outdoor Apothecary. https://www.outdoorapothecary.com/home-apothecary/

Geertsen, L. (2017, October 18). *Ayurvedic digestion tea recipe.* Empowered

References

Sustenance. https://empoweredsustenance.com/digestion-tea-recipe/

German chamomile - Uses, side effects, and more. (n.d.). WebMD. https://www.webmd.com/vitamins/ai/ingredientmono-951/german-chamomile

Gilic, V. (2023, October 23). *Growing a herb garden + health benefits of herbs.* Maple + Mango. https://www.mapleandmango.com/growing-a-herb-garden-health-benefits-of-herbs/

Gold, G. (2014, November 3). *These 7 herbs and spices can save your skin.* Everyday Health. https://www.everydayhealth.com/beauty-pictures/these-herbs-and-spices-can-save-your-skin.aspx

Green Thumb. (2021, May 5). *How to grow mint.* Green Thumb Nursery. https://www.greenthumb.com/how-to-grow-mint

Groves, M. N. (2023, March 25). *When and how to harvest herbs for medicinal use.* Hachette Book Group. https://www.hachettebookgroup.com/storey/harvest-herbs-medicinal-use/

Herb Exchange. (2022, March 25). *Your essential guide to harvesting medicinal flowers.* The Herb Exchange. https://theherbexchange.com/your-essential-guide-to-harvesting-medicinal-flowers/

Herbal gardening and its benefits. (n.d.). Comfort Keepers. https://www.comfortkeepers.com/articles/info-center/senior-independent-living/herbal-gardening-and-its-benefits/

Herbal medicine. (n.d.-a). Better Health Channel. https://www.betterhealth.vic.gov.au/health/ConditionsAndTreatments/herbal-medicine

Herbal medicine. (n.d.-b). John Hopkins Medicine. https://www.hopkinsmedicine.org/health/wellness-and-prevention/herbal-medicine

Herbalism. (2019, March 25). MentalHelp.net. https://www.mentalhelp.net/alternative-medicine/herbalism/

Hoffmaster, D. (2023, June 22). *How to make your own herbal teas.* Treehugger. https://www.treehugger.com/how-to-make-your-own-herbal-tea-recipes-and-instructions-5194393

Holy basil - Uses, side effects, and more. (n.d.). WebMD. https://www.webmd.com/vitamins/ai/ingredientmono-1101/holy-basil

Hoshaw, C. (2021, May 14). *Herbal medicine 101: How you can harness the power of healing herbs.* Healthline. https://www.healthline.com/health/herbal-medicine-101-harness-the-power-of-healing-herbs

Homemade burn salve. (2022, August 9). Our Oily House. https://www.ouroilyhouse.com/homemade-burn-salve/

How and when to harvest herbs: A one stop guide. (2023, August 8). *Grow Create Sip.* https://www.growcreatesip.com/blog/how-and-when-to-harvest-herbs-a-one-stop-guide

Iannotti, M. (2022, August 20). *How to grow and care for chamomile.* The

References

Spruce. https://www.thespruce.com/how-to-grow-chamomile-1402627

Indoor vs. outdoor plants: The differences, similarities, and how to care for both. (n.d.). Plant Shed. https://www.plantshed.com/indoor-vs-outdoor-plants-the-differences-similarities-and-how-to-care-for-both

Irene. (2019a, August 13). How to make herb-infused oils for culinary & body care use. *Mountain Rose Herbs*. https://blog.mountainroseherbs.-com/making-herbal-oils

Irene. (2019b, August 23). How to make herbal salves. *Mountain Rose Herbs*. https://blog.mountainroseherbs.com/diy-herbal-salves

James, K. (2022, April 4). *Calming tea*. Koru Nutrition Inc. https://korunutrition.com/calming-tea/

Knowles, J. (2023, September 9). *How to store herbs for culinary & medicinal purposes*. The 104 Homestead. https://104homestead.com/how-to-store-herbs/

Kruesi, G. (2023, June 30). *Herbal remedies for burns, bites, stings, and wounds*. Chelsea Green Publishing. https://www.chelseagreen.-com/2023/herbal-remedies-for-burns-bites-stings-and-wounds/

La Forge, T. (2020, April 23). *8 herbs, spices, and sweeteners that combine to activate your immune system*. Healthline. https://www.healthline.-com/health/food-nutrition/immune-system-bitters-recipe

Lapcevic, K. (2020, December 18). *4 steps to organize the herbal medicine cabinet*. Homespun Seasonal Living. https://homespunseasonalliving.-com/4-steps-to-organize-the-herbal-medicine-cabinet/

Lilly, C. (2023, October 30). *Best digestive tea recipe*. Good Food Baddie. https://goodfoodbaddie.com/best-digestive-tea-recipe/

Lockhart, B., Sharp, P., Hillock, D., Mitchell, S., & Moss, J. Q. (2020, November). *Basic plant care: Understanding your plant's needs*. Oklahoma State University Extension. https://extension.okstate.edu/fact-sheets/basic-plant-care-understanding-your-plants-needs.html

Calendula salve recipe. (2023, April 29). The Coconut Mama. https://theco-conutmama.com/calendula-salve/

Marquesen, S., & Kagan, C. (2021, August 25). *Growing, harvesting, and preserving herbs*. PennState Extension. https://extension.psu.edu/growing-harvesting-and-preserving-herbs

Marr, K. (2022, January 25). *How to make (immune-boosting) homemade elderberry syrup*. Live Simply. https://livesimply.me/immune-boosting-elderberry-syrup/

Martha Stewart Test Kitchen. (2019, January 22). *Good-digestion tea*. Martha Stewart. https://www.marthastewart.com/1155941/good-digestion-tea

Mehrabi, D. (2023, September 28). 12 of the best herbs for skin care and how

References

to use them. *BHSkin Dermatology.* https://bhskin.com/blog/12-best-herbal-skincare-products-2022/

Nebesni, J. (2019, September 19). How to make herb-infused honey + recipes. *Mountain Rose Herbs.* https://blog.mountainroseherbs.com/herbal-infused-honey

Nebesni, J. (2020, October 4). Organizing your home apothecary. *Mountain Rose Herbs.* https://blog.mountainroseherbs.com/apothecary-storage

Office of Public Outreach and Communication. (2020, April 7). *Choosing the right location for your vegetable garden.* Rutgers Newsroom. https://sebsnjaesnews.rutgers.edu/2020/04/choosing-the-right-location-for-your-vegetable-garden/

Oregano - Uses, side effects, and more. (n.d.). WebMD. https://www.webmd.com/vitamins/ai/ingredientmono-644/oregano

Osmun, R. (2023, October 26). *12 natural herbs for sleep.* EachNight. https://eachnight.com/sleep/12-natural-herbs-for-sleep/

Penrod, S. (2020, October 9). *Sweet dreams tea.* Urban Cowgirl. https://urbancowgirllife.com/sweet-dreams-tea/#mv-creation-14-jtr

Peppermint - Uses, side effects, and more. (n.d.). WebMD. https://www.webmd.com/vitamins/ai/ingredientmono-705/peppermint

Reformation Acres. (2023, November 3). *How to make an herbal burn salve.* https://www.reformationacres.com/herbal-burn-salve

Rigg, A. (2011, August 18). *Calming herbal tea.* Country Living. https://www.countryliving.com/food-drinks/recipes/a3776/calming-herbal-tea-recipe-clv0911/

Sacasas, C. (2019, February 22). *10 must-have herbs to start your own home apothecary for natural wellness.* Lone Star Botanicals. https://www.lonestarbotanicals.com/home-apothecary/

Sakawsky, A. (2022, May 15). *What to stock in a home apothecary.* The House & Homestead. https://thehouseandhomestead.com/stock-a-home-apothecary/

Silver, N. (2021, March 3). *Benefits of hydrosols.* Healthline. https://www.healthline.com/health/hydrosol

Sweetser, R. (2023, March 14). *Growing calendula: How to grow pot marigold.* The Old Farmer's Almanac. https://www.almanac.com/growing-calendula-how-grow-pot-marigold

Thomas, C. (2023, October 28). *15 medicinal herbs to grow, harvest & how to use them.* Homesteading Family. https://homesteadingfamily.com/15-medicinal-herbs-to-grow/

3 ways to preserve medicinal herbs. (2023, September 6). Serenity Hill Farmstead. https://serenityhillfarmstead.com/3-ways-to-preserve-medicinal-herbs/

References

Vinje, E. (2018, May 5). *Herbs in history*. Planet Natural. https://www.planetnatural.com/herb-gardening-guru/history/

Visser, M. (2021, September 17). *14 must-have supplies for herbalists (plus a free printable supply list)*. Herbal Academy. https://theherbalacademy.com/supplies-for-herbalists/

Wack, M. (2022, September 29). The 10 best teas for digestion. *ArtfulTea.* https://artfultea.com/blogs/wellness/9-best-teas-for-digestion

Wells, K. (2022, January 5). *How to store and organize your natural remedies*. Wellness Mama. https://wellnessmama.com/health/organize-natural-remedies/

Yi, N. (2018, August 7). *Sip on this herbal tea before, during, or after your meals to aid digestion*. POPSUGAR Fitness. https://www.popsugar.com/fitness/Digestive-Tea-Recipe-45139352

Image References

Amber, M. (2018, June 23). *Chamomile, flowers, plant image* [Image]. Pixabay. https://pixabay.com/photos/chamomile-flowers-plant-3489847/

Böckel, M. (2018, June 20). *Peppermint, green, leaves images* [Image]. Pixabay. https://pixabay.com/photos/peppermint-green-leaves-3481470/

congerdesign. (2020, June 23). *Basil bush basil, thyme, herbs image* [Image]. Pixabay. https://pixabay.com/photos/basil-bush-basil-thyme-herbs-5332038/

congerdesign. (2015, July 3). *Chamomile, camomile tea, cup image* [Image]. Pixabay. https://pixabay.com/photos/chamomile-camomile-tea-cup-gold-rim-829538/

cottonbro studio. (2020, May 28). *Photo of potted plants on wooden table* [Image]. Pexels. https://www.pexels.com/photo/photo-of-potted-plants-on-wooden-table-4503273/

Erin_Hinterland. (2020, July 2). *Cbd oil, cannabidiol, cannabinoid image* [Image]. Pixabay. https://pixabay.com/photos/cbd-oil-cannabidiol-cannabinoid-5358403/

garlandjasper. (2017, January 17). *Havana, apothecary, drugstore image* [Image]. Pixabay. https://pixabay.com/photos/havana-apothecary-drugstore-cuba-1988172/

gate74. (2017, July 19). *Tea, variety, drink image* [Image]. Pixabay. https://pixabay.com/photos/tea-variety-drink-healthy-chinese-2519551/

hajninjah. (2014, March 12). *Rosehips, berry, branch image* [Image]. Pixabay. https://pixabay.com/photos/rosehips-berry-branch-plant-red-285436/

KoolShooters. (2021, January 28). *Hanging dried green plants* [Image].

References

Pexels. https://www.pexels.com/photo/hanging-dried-green-plants-6626976/

Linde, H. (2017, August 20). *Oregano, leaves, herbs* [Image]. Pixabay. https://pixabay.com/photos/oregano-leaves-herbs-foliage-fresh-2662890/

monicore. (2017, July 7). *Spices, shelf, jar images* [Image]. Pixabay. https://pixabay.com/photos/spices-shelf-jar-kitchen-cooking-2482278/

Ortiz, M. R. (2016, July 26). *Tulsi, spice, aromatic, herb image* [Image]. Pixabay. https://pixabay.com/photos/tulsi-spice-aromatic-herb-1539181/

Pexels. (2016, November 23). *Jars, herbs, shelves images* [Image]. Pixabay. https://pixabay.com/photos/jars-herbs-shelves-store-shop-1853439/

RitaE. (2018, July 16). *Echinacea, flower, coneflower image* [Image]. Pixabay. https://pixabay.com/photos/echinacea-flower-coneflower-nature-3540788/

sergei_spas. (2019, July 16). *Flowers, flower wallpaper, calendula image* [Image]. Pixabay. https://pixabay.com/photos/flowers-calendula-yellow-flora-4340127/

Shapouri, C. (2019, Mar 28). *Person holding clear glass container* [Image]. *Unsplash.* https://unsplash.com/photos/person-holding-clear-glass-container-PwzCZVEw8vY

stux. (2017, June 19). *Spices, nature, chervil image* [Image]. Pixabay. https://pixabay.com/photos/spices-chervil-lemon-balm-chives-2419055/

Tran, V. (2019, November 23). *Photo of jar near cinnamon sticks* [Image]. Pexels. https://www.pexels.com/photo/photo-of-jar-near-cinnamon-sticks-3273989/

zerin117. (2018, May 31). *Chamomile, oil, aromatherapy image* [Image]. Pixabay. https://pixabay.com/photos/chamomile-oil-aromatherapy-herbal-3442807/